Do Clouds Rest?
Dementiadventures
with Mom

Michael Hicks

Michael Hicks

For David,

This footnote to
our lives of
shared consolations—

M

Preface

My artist mom lived her whole life in California. Well, almost. Two months before her eighty-eighth birthday my wife Pam and I made her move to Utah. Why? Her mind was cranking down. All the usual quirks of old-age-dementia: forgetting what she just said, sending the same bill payment twice, not knowing how old she was or, well, what state she lived in. The changes made her boyfriend dump her—"I can't be her caregiver"—which kept her more housebound than ever, except for the six-block walks she took every morning and afternoon, and about which she'd tell me over and over on the phone. The thought that she'd trip on one of those walks and die on the street as I sat at my office desk scared me. But what scared me more was that she still drove to the grocery store. When her license expired and the DMV wouldn't renew it and she swore to us she'd keep driving anyway, that was it. Her niece from Livermore packed her up and flew her to Utah where we got her a nice flat in the Courtyard at Jamestown, a high-end care center three blocks from where we live.

While my whole family vowed generically to attend to her and keep her happy, I decided to visit her every day for as long as she lived—weeks, months, years, who knew? She'd always been a health nut, she ate like a sparrow, and there were those daily walks. But I knew I didn't want to have to decide each day, "Do I visit or not?" So: one visit, short or long, every day.

Now and then I posted a note on Facebook about our times together so family and friends could keep up. It was a purging, a verbal exhalation. But I have to admit: it was entertainment, too. Because I saw her wit daily peeking through the haze of a fading mind. I called these postings "Dementiadventures."

Out of the blue, eight months after she moved here, she died. A friend and I gathered up my postings into a makeshift book. For some reason, one of the numbered postings was missing: there was a 40b but no 40a. When I finally found 40a in my files—it had never been posted—it seemed to hold her spirit like a genie in a bottle.

Just these two lines:

> I say to Mom, "Neat to see the clouds resting on
> the mountaintops."
> "Do clouds rest?"

And like that, she'd handed me a title.

Is there a story to go with it? Or just occasions that radiate from that question? I still can't decide.

Dementiadventure 1

The standard tests show that Mom is in steep decline. She usually doesn't know her full name, not the year, not the day of the week, not the state she lives in. She can't do simple arithmetic, can't remember all her husbands (good thing), the names of her stepchildren, and so on. And she repeats questions and observations incessantly.

But sometimes her basic stratum of wit shines through. Here are three examples of how she copes—and inadvertently helps me do the same:

1. The assessing doctor asks her if she knows what this expression means: "People in glass houses shouldn't throw stones." She says, "I don't know. I guess because they'd cut themselves."
2. I tell her for the umpteenth time that she can't have a checkbook, partly because she recently wrote a $9,800 check to someone she doesn't know for she doesn't know what. This time, she says matter-of-factly, "Well, it must have been persuasive."
3. I go to pick her up for Sunday dinner. She finds a dime on the sidewalk, hands it to me and says, "Here's your tip."

Dementiadventure 2

My dementia-beset mom continues to come off with great lines amid the dull incessant repetitions. Here are four from today:

1. After the podiatrist works on her feet for a while, she asks me what we're doing now. I say, "What do you want to do?" "I don't know," she says. "I'm free as a bird—except they don't clip birds' toenails."

2. Mom walks every morning around her building at 7:30 for exercise. After we go to the bank, our house, and a couple of stores, I say, "Well you're getting in a second walk today. Except it's not walking in a circle." She says, "Maybe my mind is."

3. At the drug store we shop for shampoo. She has no brand loyalty, can't remember any brand she's ever used. But she wants shampoo in a tube. I suggest we get a brand Pam and I use, "Bed Head." She laughs, then says, "Maybe mine should be 'Dead Head.'" (My rejoinder: "I don't think you've ever been a 'Deadhead.'" Which she wouldn't get, but you do.)

4. We get ready to curve down from the Orem, Utah bench into the Riverbottoms and I say, "Okay, this is going to feel like a big swoop." She says, "As long as something else doesn't swoop out and all over your car."

Dementiadventure 3

Explaining to my mom for the thousandth time how Pam and I are going to her house in California tomorrow to start sorting through her things for an estate sale as well as retrieving personal items of hers to bring back to Utah. And for the hundredth time she says, "I hope you don't find anything of mine that'll make you think less of me."

After giving the same placid answers again and again ("Oh, we won't look at personal things" or "We don't judge," etc.), I try a different tack.

She: I hope you don't find anything of mine that'll make you think less of me.

Me: I don't think it's possible for me to think less of you.

She: [big grin] I beg your pardon!

Dementiadventure 4

I take my mom to my school. The good news: she finds a dime on the carpet in the fifth floor E-wing hallway of the HFAC (Harris Fine Arts Center). The bad news: she keeps it in her hand and continually asks, "Where did this dime come from?"

I answer again and again, "You found it on the floor." Finally, back in the car, I say, "If you want, you can put that dime in your wallet."

She pulls her wallet from her purse but struggles to open it with just her free hand. After a minute, I point to the cup holder and say, "You can set that dime down here if you want." She waves me off, scrunches her face, and says, "Be quiet. I've got a lot of things on my mind."

"What's on your mind?"

"I'm trying to get this dime in my wallet."

"Oh," I say. "Good idea."

Dementiadventure 5

Especially when she's in front of my friends, Mom sometimes clicks into "show off" mode. Those are the fun moments.

Yesterday, at the HFAC, we're talking with Jeremy Grimshaw and I try to tell her all the things I've been working on for her when I'm not with her. "I've taken care of your Bank of America account and your Heritage Bank account, but I've still got to get your Social Security deposited to your new bank account, I've got to deal with two different Teamster incomes—Paul's pension and your supplemental benefit checks—I've got to figure out what this Franklin-Templeton thing is, you've supposedly got a Bank of America life insurance policy that they say they have no record of, and another one you listed among your assets that we're trying to locate . . ."

"Well," she says, "that's one of the benefits of getting old: your kids have to take care of that stuff for you."

"Trust me, duty's the only reason I'm doing it."

"Except you're going to get all my money."

"If you haven't spent it first."

"How do you know I haven't?"

"Of the two of us, I'm the only one that knows."

Dementiadventure 6

Three happys and a sad.

Mom's birthday is Saturday. She always asks how old she is or is going to be. After answering her truthfully (she turns 88) many times, I finally say, "You're going to be 100!"

"No way," she says. "Maybe 99."

She has had no music in her life for a couple months except the smattering of live music in the Jamestown activity room most days. So I gave her a radio tuned to Classical 89 and secured with tape so she can only adjust the volume up or down (all the way down to simulate "off"). She asks me today, "Is it okay if I leave that on all the time? It's very uplifting. And there's lots going on that downlifts me."

I come to her dinner table and she says, "This is a good time to come. I've been feeling pretty lonesome today."

So I ask her what she's doing tonight to help with that.

"Oh, there's something going on here. What's it called?" She looks at the schedule placard and points to the event. "FHE—what's that?"

"That stands for what our church calls 'family home evening.' That's a thing where people go to be lonesome together."

"Sounds good," she says.

I've played piano since junior high, seriously since high school, starting more than forty years ago. I used to play flashy hymn arrangements for her on the piano in our townhouse in Mountain View in the early '70s and for years thereafter in our house in Los Altos. She has lots of recordings of me, live and studio, playing my own music. Whenever I'd visit her through the years, she'd have me play for her. Just last week Steve Lindeman and I both played some old standards for her in Steve's office. To her delight.

Last Saturday, I take her into the activity room to check out the piano, see how it feels and if it's in tune. I start to play and she says, "I've never heard you play piano before."

I gently point out, "Oh yes, I've played for years." She keeps insisting to the contrary. I assure her that she's heard me play since I was a teenager. "You even heard me play last week at BYU," I tell her.

She disputes me. And then, in a rare moment, her eyes flashing, she pounds her fist on the piano lid and says, "I have *never* heard you play piano before in my life. I'm not that senile."

I bristle at the word. Neither of us has uttered it in the other's presence till now. But the anger, the rage in her voice and expression I know is not pointed at me but at what she knows deep down is happening to her. That's what shakes me.

When I leave her, after some words to soften the mood, I can't help but think of the ending of the great Conrad Aiken short story, "Silent Snow, Secret Snow" and I choke up:

> And with that effort, everything was solved, everything became all right: the seamless hiss advanced once more, the long white wavering lines rose and fell like enormous whispering

sea-waves, the whisper becoming louder, the laughter more numerous.

"Listen!" it said. "We'll tell you the last, most beautiful and secret story—shut your eyes—it is a very small story—a story that gets smaller and smaller—it comes inward instead of opening like a flower—it is a flower becoming a seed—a little cold seed—do you hear? we are leaning closer to you—"

The hiss was now becoming a roar—the whole world was a vast moving screen of snow—but even now it said peace, it said remoteness, it said cold, it said sleep.

Dementiadventure 7

My mom has a new friend and dinner companion: Gail. I know her name well by now because Mom introduced me at the dinner table tonight about five times. Gail is pretty lucid and, despite her quicker mind, treats Mom with patience. (She has a physical disability, yes, but I kept hearing in my head the line from Billy Joel's "Piano Man": "Man, what are *you* doing here?")

Here's a touch of Gail:

Mom: [pointing to me] This is my little boy.
Gail: Yes, she talks about you all the time.
Me: Well, she doesn't have many topics of conversation.
Gail: [smiling] I know.
I tell Gail that Mom's birthday is Saturday.
Gail: So I've heard.
Mom: [to me] So how old am I going to be?
(She's asked me that maybe fifty times in the past two weeks.)
Me: I think it's a hundred.
Mom: No way.
Me: Are you going to be ninety?
Mom: I think I'm in my nineties.
Me: No, you're actually just going to be 88.
Mom: [preening] Oh, I'm very young, then.
Gail: That's okay. A woman's not supposed to remember.

Grateful for Gail. We'll see how she holds up.

Dementiadventure 8

Shocked Mom at Day's Market scans the meat section and exclaims: "Look at all those poor animals."

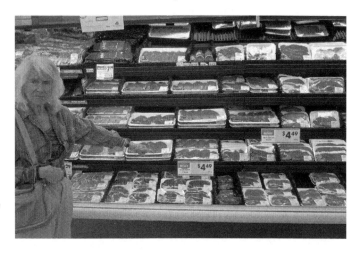

Dementiadventure 9

Mom says she's seen a few deer out on her morning walks.

I say, "You better be careful, because we've got a lot of man-eating deer around here."

"Well, I'm a woman."

She needed stamps and I thought I'd get her some funky, colorful ones that would stand out. So I got this great sheet of circus stamps. After much conversation about them, she still refuses to believe these really are stamps you can mail with. So now I'm looking for a suitable frame.

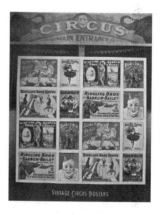

Dementiadventure 10

I'm walking with Mom around a local office building complex and point out to her this sign:

"See that?" I say. "An 'ascent advisor.' That's the guy you have to talk to before they'll let you into heaven."

"Well, what if I get to the Pearly Gates before I talk to him? What happens then?"

"What do you think?"

"I guess they'll just kick me back down. Probably to hell."

"You never know. Better make an appointment."

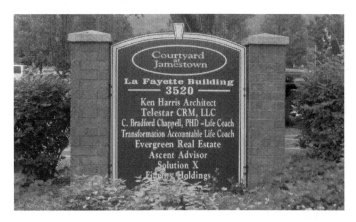

Dementiadventure 11

I go to hang some framed pictures at Mom's Jamestown apartment. She keeps telling me she doesn't want any hanging over a couch or chair where they might fall on someone.

"Well, I'm hanging them as sturdily as I can, so they shouldn't fall."

"What if we have an earthquake?"

"We don't really have those here. You're not in California anymore. And besides, you don't invite anyone in, anyway. So no potential victims."

A few more rounds of this and finally I say, "You know, God's in charge of the earthquakes, so let's hope he lays off while you're living here."

"Well, I don't want any of the pictures falling down in the middle of the night, either."

"God's in charge of all falling stuff, too, you know. If he can watch the sparrows, he can watch your pictures."

Then more about not having anything hanging over sofas or chairs. I point out that one sofa already has two constant occupants, the childhood dolls she set on it a couple of weeks ago. "Oh, you're right," I say, "Those dolls look pretty scared. So we better not hang a picture there."

I finally get one large picture hung, away from the dolls or other potential sitting places. Then we have to decide if it's straight. Don't try this with a dementia-afflicted artist. She keeps having me tap the picture an eighth-inch this way or that. (Literally: she kept saying "an eighth of an inch.") After a few minutes of this, she says, "That's good enough. I don't really invite anyone in here, anyway."

Dementiadventure 12

I showed my mom the CD *A Flintstones Motown Christmas*, thinking she'd get a laugh and maybe detect for herself the weirdness of it.

"Who are the Flintstones?" she said.

This was the scariest thing she could have said. Once a person forgets the Flintstones, one has reached the point of no return. I didn't know what to say and blurted out, "They're the modern stone-age family." I was ready to explain more, but she interrupted with, "And what's Motown?"

I paused. "Maybe this CD isn't for you."

"I do like Christmas," she said.

Dementiadventure 13

Mom's hearing continues to deteriorate, despite a hearing aid. I tell her we might need to get her a new one, though they are expensive.

"I don't want to be spending a lot on anything," she says. "'Cause I could croak any day."

"But," I say, "you want to hear it when you do."

"Not really."

I show Mom my large-print quadruple combination (all four books of Mormon scripture bound together). She's never seen one before. She noses through it and runs across a bookmark, a quarter-sheet with my picture on it advertising my April 2008 folk concert. She hands me back the book and says, "That's quite a fat bible. I'd hate to carry that one around." Pause. "Nice picture, though."

Mom tells Pam and me about her daily walk around the building and duck pond, about which she notifies us several times daily. Pam, looking for some new response, says, "Do the ducks follow you around?"

"We mingle," Mom says.

I drop Mom off at Jamestown after Sunday dinner. There's a sign over the front door that I read to her again as I drop her off: "Okay, Mom, always remember that 'Through these doors pass the finest people in the world.'"

She says, "Not until I pass through, they don't."

Dementiadventure 14

I take Mom to the BYU bookstore so she can buy some eye drops. She keeps drilling me with, "Have I ever been here before?" Each time I say, "Yes, but a long time ago." After we get her eye drops, I stroll past the "LDS History" book section and show her my books there. "You're famous!" she says. "And now I can say I'm the *mother* of the famous Michael Hicks."

A few minutes later, we walk out the doors and she asks me again, "Have I ever been here before?" Before I can answer, she answers herself, "Oh I remember. That one time when you brought me here to show me your books."

I take her by my office, outside of which is a pile of stuff I'm giving away to any takers, including a VHS of *About Schmidt*. She looks at Jack Nicholson's grizzled face on the cover and says, "Jack Nicholson? He looks like an old man."

"Well, he is an old man," I say. "But in that show he's *trying* to look like an old man."

"That's a good move," she says. "I'll have to use that line—I'm trying to look like an old lady. And they'll say, 'You're doing a hell of a job.'"

We walk out of the HFAC on the 4th floor west side. I say, "Oh, they've got some paintings on the other side. Maybe we should walk on that side."

She says, "Maybe they look better from over here."

Dementiadventure 15

I walk into Jamestown and Mom is sitting at the dining table. Her jaw drops, then she smiles and says, "I must be getting spoiled, because I hadn't seen you today and I see you every day."

"Well you're seeing me right now."

"True."

"I thought I'd take you over to our place to say 'hi' to everyone."

"Yes, but then you'd have to bring me home when we were done."

"Well, every time I take you out I have to bring you home."

"True." Points to my t-shirt. "What's that say?"

"Rick's Restoration."

"What does he restorate?"

"Antiques. Cars. All kinds of stuff."

"Does he do people?"

"Nope."

"Too bad."

Dementiadventure 16

I visit Mom every day. Every other day or every third day, I take her out somewhere, often on errands. Today I had a few, so I took her with me.

When she's meeting new people, she comes alive. When she's just with me, the conversational focus, let's say, narrows. Today, for a little over an hour, there were two topics: Mom's next-door neighbor waking up and wondering where her teeth were; and, what happened to Mom's "cut-off jeans."

Here's a slice of the conversation, highly abridged:

"You know, my next-door neighbor has been weird all day because she woke up this morning and couldn't find her teeth."

"You mean her dentures?"

"I don't know, she just said her teeth were missing."

"That's sad. She might have forgotten that her real teeth fell out a long time ago or else she misplaced her dentures overnight."

"And I can't find my cut-off jeans. Did you take them?"

"I've never seen you wear cut-off jeans. Your *regular* jeans I took home yesterday to wash them."

"I wear cut-off jeans every day of my life, except for Sundays."

"I've never seen you in cut-off jeans, just regular jeans."

"No, they only come down to here [motions to her knee]."

"They actually come to your ankle, but you do wear them every day."

"Do you know what happened to them?"

"I took them home to wash them last night."

"I sure wish I knew what happened to them."

"I'll bring them back tomorrow."

"Do you think I'm losing my mind?"

"Not your mind. But your memory, which is a big part of your mind."

"Part of the problem is that somebody took my cut-off jeans."

"I took them home to wash them and I'll bring them back tomorrow."

"So, do you think I'm weird?"

"Kind of."

"Well, I'm probably just going to get weirder and weirder."

"I'm not sure how you could be any weirder, but it's possible."

"I don't know if that's a compliment or an insult."

"Neither. It's just an observation."

"You might think I'm weird, but my neighbor's really weird. She woke up this morning and wondered where her teeth were. She thinks someone came in and stole them."

"I don't think anyone is going around breaking into people's apartments to steal teeth."

"Probably not. I just wish I knew what happened to my cut-off jeans . . . "

And so on. Multiply that by about twenty and you get why after I drop her off I switch on the car stereo and crank it up really loud.

Dementiadventure 17

The Weather Today

I pick Mom up to take her to BYU to see the latest art. She's wearing her usual double layer of fall/winter shirts. She starts to complain about the heat. I tell her it's time to start dressing like it's summer. "You see, in Utah we're in the desert. It's hot in summer and cold in winter. And not much in between. It's like Jesus. Hot or cold. Remember how he said, 'Ye are neither hot nor cold. Ye are just lukewarm. So I will spew thee out of my mouth'"?

"Jesus said that?"

"He did."

"That wasn't a very nice thing to say, Jesus."

"Anyway, the days are going to be pretty long for awhile. Lots of summer sun. You know, yesterday was the longest day of the year."

"It was?"

"It was."

"Well, I hope it was a good one, then. Because I don't remember it."

Dementiadventure 18

The Truth About Focus

I get in the car to pick up Mom at quarter to 2. I turn on the CD player to Madonna's *Bedtime Stories* and the smooth-jam first track, "Survival," starts up:

> I'll never be an angel
> I'll never be a saint, it's true
> I'm too busy surviving

Madonna's producers scattered digital pops and clicks around the album to mimic an old record, a genre with which I've spent lots of my life. One of the things that made CDs seem better than records was that records wore down and got scratched, sometimes enough to make the needle get stuck on the vinyl. When that happened the record kept repeating the same few seconds of music until you came and pushed the needle across the scratch and the music skipped ahead.

Since artists know how to exploit dysfunction, what was a flaw (getting stuck) eventually became a new motivic device—the loop. Madonna uses them. Phil Glass uses them. I even use them. A few seconds of music that keep recurring. In the old days they'd call that ostinato—the Italian cognate for "obstinate." Stubborn.

Mom is stubborn. Always has been. But when she loops now, which is all the time, it's not stubbornness. It's the needle getting stuck in her brain. Today she asks me over and over how many copies my latest book has sold. I've learned the routine that works for both of us. I give her a slightly different answer each time. Because I'm not ready to loop with her. Not entirely. I have to keep my mind swerving enough for sanity. Whatever sales figure I give her, she gets excited. And then she asks me again. It's like playing catch with a puppy. No point insisting that she remember what you just told her. And no point getting mad. It's got to be variations on a theme, for both our sakes.

I take her to my office at BYU, where I have to pick a few things up and leave a few things behind. (That's my routine.) I have walls of books and a thousand trinkets and oddities in the office. She sits down in front of one shelf and pulls out George Antheil's book *Bad Boy of Music*. She flips through the pages for a minute, then puts it back on the shelf. Then she pulls out the anthology *Artists as Professors*. She flips through the pages, then puts it back. I wonder what she'll choose next. She stares, her eyes move across the shelf and she pulls out . . . *Bad Boy of Music*. Flips through it, then returns it. What next? *Artists as Professors*. And on and on.

I try so hard each day to learn to focus. My mind is a freeway. I keep crossing the lanes, cutting in and out. I try little exercises to stay on track. I work on ways to slow down and stay in the same lane. But when I see focus turn mandatory, as I see happening in her, I want to step on the accelerator pedal in my head and jerk the steering wheel.

Stubbornness, steadfastness, determination, doggedness: all those versions of focus can reward us or damn us, I guess. But they make the world turn. Great minds have to focus. Great machinery has to loop. But when a record gets stuck, it's not that. You can pretend it's a loop, as I try to do with Mom each day and just ride it like a Madonna groove. But no true focus is mandatory. And no mandatory focus is true. That's what I feel, at least, when I see her mind turning into a broken record. I try to push each little ostinato dialogue across the scratch with some thought or joke or even challenge, which works for a minute or two. Maybe longer. And then the needle gets stuck again. I offer her another book to look at, but soon it's back to *Bad Boy of Music* and *Artists as Professors*.

After a half-hour at BYU, I drive back from campus and drop her off back at Jamestown. She thanks me, as always, for taking her out for awhile. She closes the door, waves, and walks back inside. I turn up the car stereo, as I do after every visit, trying to blast the rhythm of her word loops out of my head and disgorge the image of her picking up the same two books over and over. Madonna goes into her own loop, and I sing along, loudly:

> Up and down and all around
> It's all about survival
> Up and down and all around
> It's all about survival
> Up and down and all around
> It's all about survival
>
> Up and down and all around
> It's all about survival
> Up and down and all around . . .
> (fadeout)

Dementiadventure 19

I take Mom some snapshots of her and her four(!) different boyfriends from 1972. I can only remember two of the guys, though know the names of three of them, and, in any case, want to see if the pictures would jog any memories for her, hopefully pleasant ones.

She vaguely remembers two of their faces, especially after I coach her on who they were—one of them, Wally, she'd actually been planning to marry back in the day. After talking through all this as much as we can, always elliptically, she says, "Now these were all before I had you, right?"

"No," I say, "I was sixteen at the time."

"Oh, Jesus," she says.

Dementiadventure 20

It's Fourth of July. I pick up Mom in the afternoon and she begins a continuous loop of how "It was a weird day," because they moved her regular table in the dining room and she had to sit at another one with "a lady who was about a hundred years old." This is the mantra of the hour. I nod a lot.

I drive her a few places, including the Provo River and the ritzy Stonegate neighborhood, where our bishop lives. There we get out of the car and walk along the river, talk about the snowfall runoff and how big the houses are on this street. As we drive away from Stonegate, we pass a huge new set of buildings on the left that are meant to rival her home, Jamestown. I point out the big sign on the front of the place. She reads it aloud: "'Assisted Living and Memory Care.' I guess that's because they have so many old people around here who are losing their memories. [Pause] I have a great memory!" Then, looking at me and smiling, "What was your name again, dear?"

As I drop her off, I point out how much nicer her place looks than the would-be competitor down the road. "That other one kind of looks like a prison," I say.

"Well this one's kind of a prison, too," she says. "I can't get out, except when some nice person like you takes me out. But today was a weird day. They moved the table where I usually sit and I had to sit with this lady who looks like she's a hundred years old."

"See you tomorrow," I say.

Dementiadventure 21

On her tabletop at Jamestown, Mom has an 8″×10″ black and white photo of her and her high school sweetheart, Jim Barmore. It was taken soon before he entered the U.S. Navy during the last year of World War II. They'd been an item since she was fifteen and planned to marry, but for reasons I still don't know, broke up after he came home from the war. He married someone else from her hometown of Santa Paula, became a police officer there, and was killed in the line of duty in 1953. The city built a monument to him outside the police station in 1988. Jim's son and even grandson both became policemen, too, and last month I sent them all the photos Mom had of Jim that she wasn't in, many of them taken on the ship where he was stationed. The family immediately knew who I was because they all knew about Marilyn. What they knew, I don't know, but her presence in their collective memory seems as vivid as his is in her fading mind. The 8″×10″ Navy service photo I sent to his family is inscribed, "Remember me always, Jim."

The photo here, taken yesterday, shows her bony finger pointing to one random diary entry (4 April 1945). I had her put her finger there so you could see how tiny her handwriting was in the five-year diary she kept back then. I don't know if I'll ever have the time or patience—or eyesight—to read through her diaries, which she still keeps, mostly on post-it notes stuck in her nightstand drawer. But even this one entry cast me back

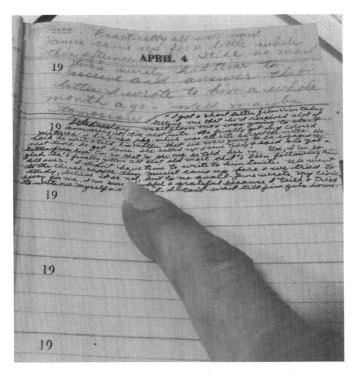

into the heart of a seventeen-year old Presbyterian girl trying
to keep ties with her Navy man—and cheating in her civics class.

I got a short letter from Jim today telling me
that he'd received alot of mail from me + was
going to start answering it the next nite. He
finally got my colored pictures + his Xmas pack-
age which was all rite except the nuts. He said he
wrote + told his mother that we were going to be
engaged the next time he got home. She called
up + came today + said she got a letter from him
too so that is the one he told her in. Gee, I'm
so glad he's finally gotten all that old mail that's

been following him all over. I didn't have time to write to him tonite. We went to the church supper then Muriel came up here + we tried to study, believe it or not, but to no avail. June* wrote my civics essay for me. I'm sure thankful + grateful because I tried + tried to write one myself + couldn't do it. I can't wait till Jim gets home.

---

* Mom's older sister

Dementiadventure 22

Mom didn't want to come to Johnny's wedding and that was fine with us—too confusing for her and fatiguing for us. But she talked about it for many days beforehand, always the same few words and questions. From the verbal haze emerged a few quotables.

She kept asking me if I was going to the wedding. I always said yes, until one time I say, "It's my *son's* wedding, so, obviously I'm going."

"When it's over you'll be glad you did," she says.

She sees me in my suit when I visit her before the wedding reception. She looks me over and says, "You look so . . . uh . . . priestly."

When I bring her to our house on Sunday, she asks many times how the wedding went. I show her lots of pictures and we talk about them. As I take her home, she tells me how nice it is to have people taking care of her meals and entertainment and so forth—the privilege of being old, she says.

I reply, "Then I'm not going to call it your 'home' or your 'apartment' any more. I'm going to call it your 'estate.' You know, since you're treated like a queen there. And should be, of course."

"Well," she says, "the woman who *is* the queen of the place now—I wouldn't want to be her."

Dementiadventure 23

I pick up Mom to take her to Harmon's. She needs deodorant. She shows me her used-up stick.

I say, "This says 'Regular Scent.' Is that how you want to smell—regular?"

"Better than smelling irregular," she says.

She shows me today's schedule of activities. "This morning they had a 'hearing screening,'" she says.

"Did you go?"

"I don't need anyone to tell me I can't hear. I can tell *them* that."

She buys make-up. "I need this to make me beautiful," she says. "Or make me *try* to be beautiful." Pause. "Possibly."

At Harmon's she sees the "Naked" brand of drinks and asks, "Why do they call it 'Naked'?"

"I don't know."

"Maybe you have to be naked to buy it."

Dementiadventure 24

My mom kept for herself only one painting by her mother: this one, called "The Patriarch." It hangs next to her bed at Jamestown and whenever I see it, I see a human brain, the stem and blood vessels and the light shining in the midst of it. I never saw it that way till it hung over Mom's nightstand these last months.

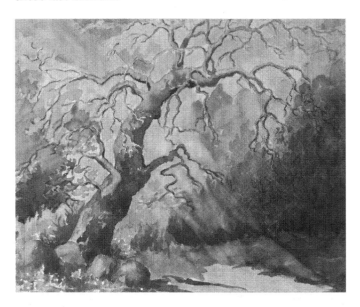

Today I took Mom a large print of this photo I found of her mother at the painting's first exhibit (Santa Paula High School, date unknown). The man with her mom in this photo is Douglas Shiveley, probably the best known of the Ventura County circle of artists that included Mom's mom. Mom loved getting the print of this picture and, though she can't remember from one sentence to the next most of the time, can't remember even her three husbands without a lot of coaching, looked at this picture and said, "That's Douglas Shiveley with her, isn't it?"

Light still hangs in the branches.

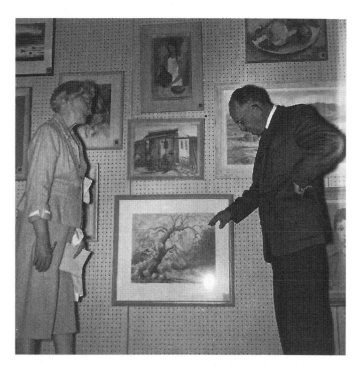

Dementiadventure 25

Soundtrack Edition

They say playing piano is like riding a bike. But my mom hasn't ridden a bike or played the piano in many years. So at my office last week I invite her to sit down at the piano and see if she can still manage.

She opens the hymnbook to "I Need Thee Every Hour" and starts to play. I can tell that deep down she thinks like a pianist because she gratuitously arpeggiates and throws in some extra bass octaves in the left hand. But her first time through the hymn she has Ivesian moments I'm sure she doesn't intend (though I like 'em!).

Then, with not a beat to spare, she starts into the second verse. She's confident and focused. A much cleaner rendition this time. And she knows it. Twice is enough to prove that to herself, so she stops.

I've gotten her some sheet music of religious songs I know she likes and urged her to practice at the piano where she lives. But I somehow know she won't.

I myself never play for her anymore, because every time I do, she insists she's never heard me play piano before, ever. And I, who've played for and around her for forty-nine years, can't take the chips in my identity. I get enough of those already, as she daily, though unwittingly, compensates for the huge chunks breaking off from her own.

Dementiadventure 25a
(supplemental)

Last time I said I wouldn't play piano for Mom anymore because, when I do, she always insists she's never heard me play before. Today I bring her to my BYU office, have to run two quick errands, and tell her to play my piano while I'm gone.

"I don't think I remember how to play piano," she says.

"Oh, yes you can. You played just the other day."

"What should I play?"

"Just grab the hymnbook and see what you can play." Then I leave.

I come back in ten minutes and hear her playing through the office door. She's doing well. I come in and she stops. I decide to go ahead and play, too, no matter what she says. She needs to always know that part of me, I think, if she's going to know me at all. Most self-censorship stinks, anyway. And I even have this thought that her own playing just now has freed up her mind, her powers of recall.

So I sit down and start playing, by heart, my own personal bossa nova medley of "Wave" and "Night and Day." I play them as furiously as I can, with all the stops pulled out—as many notes in as many registers as I can muster (and a few I can't) to dazzle her. That way, maybe she won't say anything.

But she does. Two things, over and over.

"You're self-taught, aren't you?"

"Yes."

And, "Do you play by ear or do you read music?"

"Both."

A good day at the keys.

Dementiadventure 26

I go see Mom and she's sitting with her friend Gail at the dinner table. Here's some of the conversation, with repetitions and most of Gail's comments left out.

Mom asks about the printed schedule for the day. "What's this 'Meet the Candidates' thing? Candidates for what?"

"Those are candidates for Provo city council coming to talk about themselves."

"Why should I go to that? I'm not going to be voting for any of them."

"Yeah, but they don't know that. So you go and meet them and act interested and they'll . . . "

"Butter me up."

"Right."

Gail says she went to the temple today. Mom says to me, "I didn't go, though."

"Well, they wouldn't let you in, anyway. You'd be sitting in a hot bus for two hours."

"Then I don't want to go."

We talk about what day of the week it is and she asks me for the third time, "Did you bring my clean laundry to my room?"

"Yeah. Oh, but I saw some folded laundry on your bed. Is that stuff you hand washed?"

"I think that's my pajamas."

"So did you wash them yourself?"

"I can't say they're immaculate. But I'm not sleeping with anyone, so it doesn't matter if I smell like a skunk."

"But you don't want to be attracting the skunks."

Mom tells Gail, "I don't know if I've introduced you to my son. This is Mike. Mikey."

Gail nods, grins, and says, "Yes, we've met."

"Mikey Hicks," Mom says.

"Oh," Gail says, "I don't know that I ever knew your last name, Marilyn."

"Well, she's added a couple since she and I had the same one. But she's gone by Marilyn Thompson for the past thirty-five years or so."

While I'm saying that Mom says, "It's Marilyn Webster." I correct her and she says "What are those other names? I don't remember them."

"You're actually Marilyn Webster. Hicks. Gray. Thompson."

She scrunches her face, looks at Gail and says, "I get around."

Dementiadventure 27

Mom complains a lot about the temperature. It's always either too hot or too cold—often within seconds of one another. I go to get her at Jamestown: she's in her jacket, says it's too cold in there. She walks outside: takes the jacket off, too hot. I put her in my car and turn on the air conditioner: within ten seconds it's, when is this thing going to start working? Within thirty seconds: awfully cold in here! Parking lot at BYU, she gets out and complains about the heat. We get ten seconds into the shade and she's too cold. Etc.

As we leave BYU, this continues and in quiet exasperation I say, "Let's see if you can go thirty seconds without complaining."

"That's what women are for," she says.

"Complaining?"

"Complaining about the men they're with."

Dementiadventure 28

Buying a birthday card with Mom to give to my son Johnny and she keeps saying "I don't really know him" and "He won't know who I am" and I keep telling her that she might not remember but he's 24 and he's known her since he was born and I try to explain that her memory is going and when she finally picks out a card she says the same things again and I give her a pen to sign it and she asks "How do I sign it—Aunt Marilyn?" and I say "You're not his aunt, he's your grandson" and she asks me this again and so I help her to sign "Grandma Thompson" though she keeps insisting he won't know who she is and I assure her that he will and on the way home she says "This is a transitional time for me—at some point I might not even know my own name" and I say "You won't but I will" and she says "Thank you."

Dementiadventure 29

The Persistence of Memory: Grades

Mom won't hang any of her art on the wall except this drawing of the house she lived in at San Jose State in the mid-1940s (right). Why? Because, as she points out every time I'm at her place, she got an A+ on it in her drawing class. It's the only A+ she ever got and she measures the value of the work on that one grade. So other, far more accomplished works of hers sit in the corner (below).

So remember, you who grade: that grade—good or ill—may be one of the last things someone will forget.

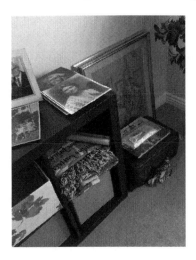

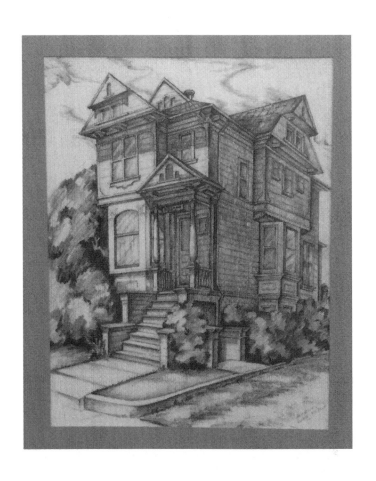

Dementiadventure 30

I often wonder what Mom does each day. "Oh, I'm very busy," she usually says when I ask her, but she can't recall a thing she's done. I looked in her bathroom yesterday and saw the sink and got some idea.

"This must take some time," I said, "to keep this so neat."

"Oh, it's a mess," she said.

"But you've got everything laid out very carefully."

"That's just for my morning ritual."

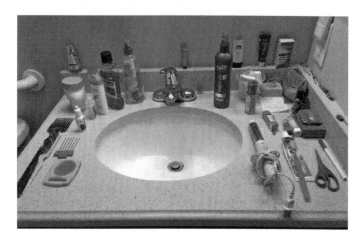

Dementiadventure 31

Mom and her sister both have dementia. When they write letters to each other, I cringe and grin at the same time:

June writes: "I'm living in Vista Cove, in Arcadia. Its a nice place + I get all my meals. . . . [three sentences later:] I'm in good health and glad of it. This place is called Vista Cove in Arcadia. We get good meals here. . . . [three sentences later] But am glad to be in good health." Etc.

Still: I do love the exclamation points! They show a positive frame of mind!

Plus: lots of love and longing in each line.

(!!!)

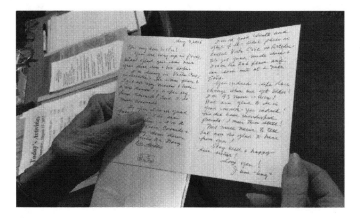

Dementiadventure 32

Every time I go outside with Mom, every single time for months now, she always says at least once, "Look at that beautiful cloud."

And I say to myself, "Let that be a lesson to you."

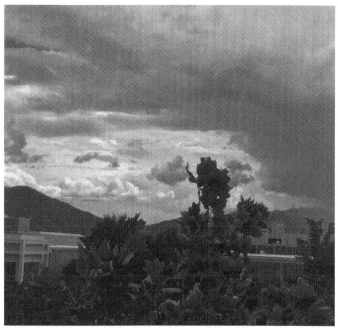

Last week outside my office window.

Dementiadventure 33

Another Thursday (Abridged Version)

I knock on Mom's door. She opens it. It's very dark, as usual. She thanks me for coming. "You've brightened my day," she says.

I flip on two light switches. "There, now I've really brightened your day."

"That's *too* bright," she says.

I drive her to BYU just to get her out and about. As we drive away, she says, "Thanks, you've rescued me."

"Not much," I say.

"Okay, rescued *temporarily*."

She asks me often about the haze on the mountains. I tell her it's smoke from California wildfires, Most of the time she laughs and says, "I doubt that." One time she says, "Where'd you hear that—in the *newspapers*?" Then she asks me why she can't smell the smoke.

"It's faint," I say, "but you don't smell as well as you used to."

"Oh, so you're saying I stink?"

At BYU she keeps asking, "What day is it today?"

I keep telling her, "It's Thursday."

One time, she retorts, "Well, I'll be darned."

On the drive home she says, "I don't think I could find my way around here."

I say, "I don't think you could find your way out of the parking lot."

She chuckles and says, "True. Old people have a way of getting lost."

I drop her back at Jamestown. "You're doing something very important here by taking me out so I don't feel like an inmate."

"Thanks. Even though you are."

"I know, but don't remind me."

Dementiadventure 33a
(supplemental)

Mom and I are talking about her first car, a '34 Ford, and she wonders whatever happened to it.

"Could be anything from being scrapped to being restored," I say.

"It'd probably be worth some money now."

"No doubt."

Then we talk about her old dolls, now sitting on one of her easy chairs and she says they're probably worth a lot of money and I agree and then she says:

"Anything old is worth something except humans."

Dementiadventure 34

Mom's started asking if I was adopted, because she doesn't remember giving birth to me or when I became her son.

Dementiadventure 35

Illustrated

1. I pick Mom up to take her for a visit to BYU. I ask if she wants to throw out any of the daily or monthly schedules she's gotten since she moved here in March. "No. I might need to refer back to something." (Like mother, like son! But even I'm more ruthless with paper than she.)

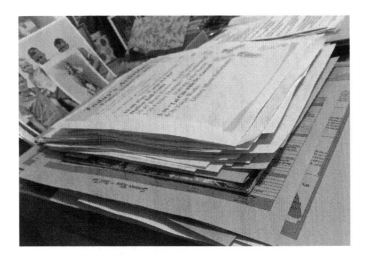

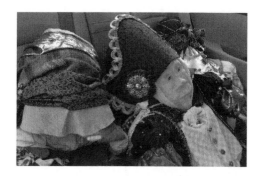

2. I've had these rare James Christensen "Voyage of the Basset" handmade figures in the back seat of my car for a few weeks, hoping to sell them to . . . I don't know who. Every time I pick Mom up she asks about them, mostly if they're still there, if they have names, etc. Today she gives her best line: "What are these—your bodyguards or something?"

3. She is quite upset about how this guest artist spells her name.

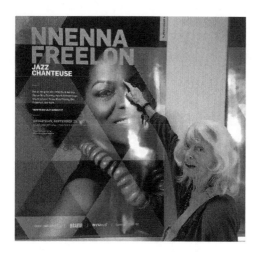

4. She always talks about the beauty of our Utah clouds. Today we have lots of jet trails in the sky, much to her delight. As for the dismal reconstruction of our parking lots and the blocking of roads around the Fine Arts Center, though, she offers this gem: "I thought smart people ran universities."

Aside from such moments, lots of grinding repetition and exercises in patience and loss—as when I sing "A Foggy Day" for her at the piano and she says, "I've never heard you play and sing at the same time."

"I have since I was a boy and all through my teenage and college years," I say, with disappointment.

"But not at home," she says.

"Usually at home," I say. "You weren't there a lot, though. So that's part of it. But mostly you've just forgotten those years of our lives." She nods, a puzzled look on her face. Her consolation: she's learned to accept the verdict. My consolation: I like that she remembers she's heard me play the piano at all, which usually she doesn't. I can let the singing part slide.

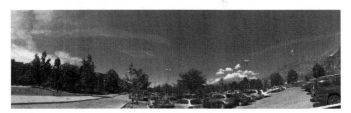

Dementiadventure 35a

At Jamestown . . .

    Mom: This must be a really boring place.

    Me: Why?

    Mom: I can't remember a thing I did today.

Dementiadventure 36

Whenever I take Mom to the store she says, over and over, "I'm sure when I get home I'll remember something I was supposed to get at the store." I have various ways of answering her and I've learned to always check all her cupboards and shelves and countertops before going to the store so we can verify that there was nothing she needed. Still she repeats this mantra every time we go shopping. Even though it can be grating, I try to get her out of the house as much as possible and that often means having her go to the store with me.

Today, I try a new tack. After checking all the usual places in her apartment, I say, "Okay, I'll take you to the store with me as long as you don't say you're sure when you get home you'll remember something you were supposed to get at the store. We just checked and there's nothing. So I don't want you to say that today."

"Okay, I'll just think it."

She says it three times before we get to the car. I hold up three fingers and say, "Now, that's three times already you've said that thing you said you weren't going to say."

"I thought that was just at the store," she says.

As we drive, she says it twice more, I hold up five fingers and say, "That's five times you've said that thing you said you wouldn't."

"It's just something I say. And that you notice tells me how well you know me."

A minute later she says it again. I tell her that's six times. She says, "I know, I'm getting dumb."

"That's not dumb. That's just forgetting things. That's not the same as dumb."

"I'm really old, you know."

"Tell me about it," I say and she laughs.

"My forgetting is just elderly symptoms."

"That's a good way to put it."

We park at Harmon's, walk into the store and she says that thing before we get twenty feet inside. I say, "That's seven times you've said that thing you weren't going to say."

She looks me straight in the eye and says, "I'm just *emphasizing*."

Dementiadventure 36a
(supplemental)

Mom was fascinated—and scared—by this display at Harmon's. She had no interest in what it meant. (Logos of the rival schools BYU and University of Utah, the boxes surrounding the Y in blue and those surrounding the U in red.) A California girl, she was sure it would collapse in our next earthquake.

So there's your update: rivalry can kill.

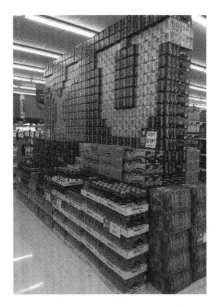

Dementiadventure 36b
(supplemental)

At the store again today with Mom. She started up as usual saying, "I know once I get home I'll remember what I needed to get at the store."

I pointed to this shelf and said, "Well, it doesn't matter, because, as you can see, it's sold out."

"But what was it that sold out?"

"How should I know? *You're* the one that wanted it."

And she never brought it up again.

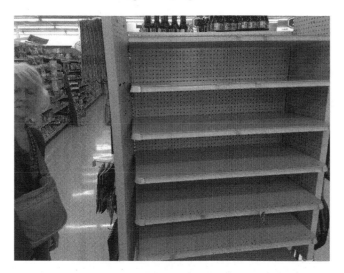

Dementiadventure 37

As I mentioned, for a month I've had these large James Christensen figures in the back seat of my car, trying to figure out what to do with them. (I'm out of garage space.)

Meanwhile, my mom is out of lipstick. "I mostly need it in case I got out for dinner," she says.

"You basically go in for dinner anymore."

"But what if I get a hot date?"

"I wouldn't be looking for one around here [at the assisted living center]," I say.

"What about my boyfriends in your back seat?"

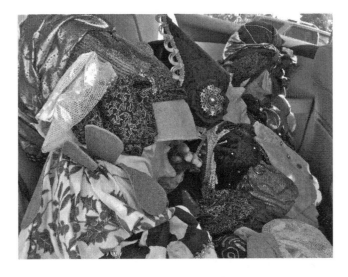

Dementiadventure 38

How can I help you understand? I put it like this to Pamela today: Imagine the movie *Groundhog Day*, but it keeps restarting not after a day but after 30 to 60 seconds. *Groundhog Minute*. That's what most visits with Mom have become. I like to get her out of the house for a ride just to hear her respond to the clouds or an odd car or a street closure, but mostly to keep sensory input beyond repetitions of questions and comments streaming into my patient but exhausted brain.

The clever bon mots become less and less frequent as her brain struggles like a beetle under a hatpin to survive, cope, proceed. The exceptions come like gentle flickers in a cave. Such as:

"I can't stay long," I say. "I've got some groceries in the trunk I've got to get home and get them into the fridge."

"What kind of groceries?"

"Some milk and some yogurt."

"Well, if it was ice cream I could see it."

Meanwhile, she tried to play piano again a couple weeks ago and the decline had steepened. Whereas before, she could keep the music bumpy but steady, like a Disneyland car running on a track, now she slid off the road in ways that were somewhere between Charles Ives and *Carnival of Souls*. She'd flip through the hymnbook, play a hymn, "Rock of Ages." But her fingers lost their way and performed the "right" fingering on the wrong keys. Modes shifted, keys jerked. She kept playing, not a moment's notice of what had happened—or perhaps a perverse pleasure in the novelty. But no recognition in her face, just a typist's confidence with random phonemes emerging.

She'd go to another, "Silent Night." Same thing. Then she'd flip through the book and arrive at . . . "Rock of Ages." Same thing as before—in principle, though not in detail. Unaccountable variations on a theme. She'd flip through pages again and arrive at "Silent Night." And on and on, with "I Need Thee Every Hour" soon thrown into the rotation. Three songs around and around for twenty minutes, each time seemingly chosen via browsing, and each time with the fingers losing place as though one had shaken a bookmark out of a book and reinserted it somewhere vaguely near where it had been before.

Music. You can't live with it and you can'y kufe ;oqothuo mbf7e*^.

Dementiadventure 39

Mom's Biggest Laugh

She doesn't much, though giggles a lot. Today: the biggest, heartiest laugh I've heard from her in six months.

I visit her at 4. She tells me over and over what a "weird day" it's been. I ask her why and what she did today.

"I can't remember," she keeps answering.

"Maybe what's weird about it is you can't remember. That's kinda weird."

"I don't know. It's just been a really weird day. You're the only un-weird thing about it."

"That's good—but sad."

"It's just been a weird day! But you're the best thing that's happened to me today."

"That is sad."

"That should make you happy."

"Why?"

"Because you're the best thing that's happened to me today."

"But that's sad."

"Why is that sad?"

"That I'm the best thing that's happened to you today."

And she laughed and laughed. The lesson? A well-placed repetition in the right context can make all the difference. Or, as they say: timing is everything.

Dementiadventure 40

I played and sang Monday night at Jamestown. "Brigham Young Songs." The posters had my mom confused for three days ahead. "Where is this being held?" she asked me again and again. Right here, in the events room, I told her.

"How will I get there?"

"You'll be there already, it's right next to the room you eat in, where all your programs are."

"Will I see you after your show is finished?"

"You'll see me while I'm doing it."

"Can I come to your show?"

"Just walk down from your room."

"Where is it being held?"

Etc.

Things got worse. My doing this show unnerved her more than I could have known.

As I was setting up, she asked me repeatedly why I was there. Didn't I have a show? Where is it going to be? As other people came in the room, one woman kept telling her to sit in the front row. She insisted not. "I don't sit in the front row."

"But you're a guest of honor."

"Why?"

"Because this is your son."

She laughed and said, "This is my little boy," as she always says. But she kept moving to the middle of the room, where she always sits. The woman would not let her.

"You must sit in the front row. You're a guest of honor."

"Why?"

Etc.

At the end of the concert, she stood up and started pacing, asking Pam how she was going to get home. Pam kept assuring her that this is where she lives. She came up and asked me if I'd be staying at her house. Soon it was clear that she thought this venue was near her house in Los Altos and we'd come there to visit. She got more and more flustered about how she was going to get home, or, if she was home, as we told her, where we were going to stay. She started saying, as she says more and more these days, "I'm all messed up." We finally persuaded her back to her room. As she left, she said "I'm all messed up" again. And this one new thing—never heard or even implied by her before in my hearing: "I guess my little boy is all grown up."

It was a thrill to have so many people getting the humor of some songs. But sad to know my mom knew nothing about even what was happening or why I was there doing this. Or why she was sitting in the front row. Or why anyone would be laughing.

Dementiadventure 40a

I say to Mom, "Neat to see the clouds resting on the mountaintops."

"Do clouds rest?"

Dementiadventure 40b

As I drive Mom around, we often pass this street sign. Today she remarks on it for the first time.

"Sounds ominous," she says.

"Why?"

"It's like you're going to jail or something."

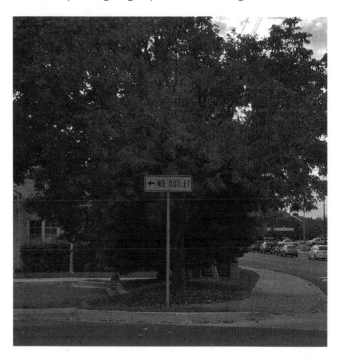

Dementiadventure 40c

My Non-Mormon Mom Reviews Mormon
General Conference

She went to the big-screen showing of General Conference this morning at Jamestown. Her one-word review: "Arduous."

More: "They kept showing this movie all the time and there were all these people in it I didn't know and they kept saying things I didn't understand so I left."

Dementiadventure 41

I'm just shy of visiting my mom every day for seven months.* Have I learned anything? I don't know. Mostly a bunch of clichés. Here are three.

1. "Eighty percent of success is showing up."** Mom knows when I'm there. She doesn't remember if I've been there. And she doesn't know if I'll be there again. But I remember. I know. So showing up is my job. Being faithful trumps being useful. She took me by the shoulders the other day and said: "I don't care if you're just here for a few minutes or a long time. You need to know it always makes me happy that you came." She's accepted now that she doesn't know how long I've been there or when I was last there, a month ago or an hour ago. I've learned to forget the grand plan and show up each day. Because it's all "line upon line," as the scripture says. Or as she learned doing crosshatching on a lifetime of drawings.

2. "If you tell the truth you don't have to have a good memory."*** I love how every time we go outside she says how beautiful the clouds are. Or how

lonely a cloud looks if it's the only one. Or how ominous storm clouds look. Or how one side of the sky differs from another side. Most of the time she points up the moment we walk out the door. And I think: that's truth, that's honest, that's right. She doesn't have to lie anymore. She doesn't even get to. She responds from the heart to the beauty all around. I find myself stopping more often when I'm walking alone and scanning the skies, the mountains, the trees. More important, I guess, I worry less and less about fitting what I say now to what I may have said back then. I just try to observe with a fresh eye and say what I think. We're all just clouds, anyway. As she's helped me learn.

3. "The show must go on."***** Whenever I knock on her door I think: someday, maybe today, I'll knock and she won't answer, but she'll be inside, not sleeping, not deaf, just gone. But till then her show and my show and all of our shows have to go on. I have an old friend who lives near her at Jamestown. Walter. He is a magician. He's been doing tricks and illusions his whole life. And Walter did a show for the Jamestown residents the other day. I don't know if many of them even knew what it was to be fooled anymore, or if they could recall what he showed them when each trick started all the way to when it ended. But, I thought, he did the show, because that's what

he does. And they came because that's what they do. And I thought, how beautiful that he knew, "I can still do this," and they felt, "This is happening and I want to be there." I want to be like him and like them, both, sure that the show must go on in this endless, beautiful set of illusions, whether we're still fooled or not.

Dementiadventure 42

Today I was driving Mom around and we passed an art supply store.

"That's where you'd be hanging out back when you were still doing art."

"Art supplies? I have plenty of those."

"Actually you don't anymore. But you don't need them because you don't do art now."

"True. I spent my whole life doing art. I used to do all the artwork for HP. Hewlett-Packard. But now I'm all arted out."

Dementiadventure 42a
(supplemental)

Every time we shop, my mom wants the smallest size of every-thing, on the pretext that "I won't live long enough to use that much" of a larger size.

Today, she was almost out of her Pond's cold cream, of which she always gets the same medium size jar. "Let's get you another one of these," I said.

"Oh, no, I won't live long enough to use that much."

"I think you will, even though you always say you won't. But maybe that's up to you."

"No, it's not up to me. It's up to the Lord."

"Well, you're in luck then, because the Lord told me he wouldn't take you before you finished your next jar of cold cream."

"Oh. Okay."

Dementiadventure 43

Mom stood frozen with fear at the giant spiders hanging in webs above the produce section at Harmon's. But, as an artist, she took delight in the children's painted pumpkins by the pharmacy.

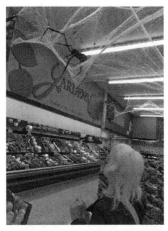

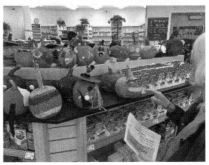

Dementiadventure 44

I walk in to Jamestown this afternoon and Mom is sitting at her table in the dining room.

"You're here early," I say.

"I don't know what time it is or what day it is or what I did today or if it's lunch or dinner or if I've ordered yet or where I'm living. I guess I'm starting to realize I'm an old lady."

"Well, you are, that's true. Do you still draw?"

"Yeah, I can draw."

"Why don't you start drawing things and people around here?"

"I have to be *inspired*."

Dementiadventure 45

I'm leaving Mom's apartment and she asks what I'm doing tonight.

"I'm going home to eat dinner and watch the Republican presidential debate."

"I don't really watch much anymore." She points to the corner and says, "I've probably only turned on the TV once since I've lived here."

She doesn't have a TV.

Dementiadventure 46

See the giant spider hanging from the banister when you enter Jamestown. Some residents think it's cute. But not all.

In other news, I took Mom out for a drive today and realized I'm glad she's losing her hearing. That way she can't hear some of the things I say when I'm driving.

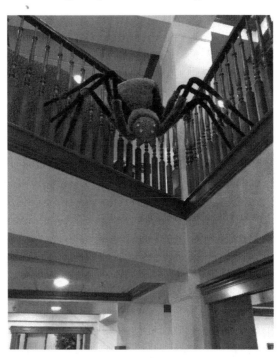

Dementiadventure 47

I stop by Mom's place at 9:30 this morning. I'm still trying to figure out what she does in the mornings. I knock. No answer. I unlock the door and let myself in. The lights are all out, the blinds drawn. I look in her bedroom and she is standing motionless at the foot of her bed, staring at the bedspread.

I watch for a few seconds, then say "Hi."

She turns and walks towards me, a worried look on her face. "Oh, hi dear. I'm all messed up today." (Something she says every day now.) "I'm feeling kind of weird. I can't explain it. I think I'm losing my mind or something. It's like I'm having a bad dream and I can't wake up. But I know I'm awake. What day is today?"

"Thursday." And I take her through the weekly calendar I made for her.

"I'm all messed up. It's like I've lived my whole life on another planet and now I'm on this one. Did I see you yesterday?"

"Yes. I took you for a drive, we looked at the Thanksgiving decorations around the neighborhood."

She nods tentatively. "Yes, I remember that. But something terrible's happened. I can't explain it. I'm worried I'm losing my mind. Have you noticed that happening to me lately?"

"Well, you're forgetting. That's been happening for a while now. It's just a part of your getting older."

"I can't explain it. It's something happening up here," she says, tapping the left side of her head. "I just hope I can get back to normal again someday."

"What does it feel like right now?"

"It's like I already lived today yesterday."

Dementiadventure 48

Me: What did you do today?

Mom: I'm sure it wasn't very interesting even if I could remember it.

I take her out for a drive and for twenty minutes she points out every patch of blue sky she sees.

Dementiadventure 49

I sit down at Mom's table in the Jamestown dining room last night. I sit next to her.

"You can sit across from me, if you want," she says.

"I don't want to have to shout for you to hear me."

"Depends on what you're shouting."

Dementiadventure 50

The Good

For the first time, I took Mom to a store and she never mentioned how she'd remember things she needed once she got home. She usually says some variant of that at least five times every trip. Not a peep about it today.

The Bad

She couldn't think about what she needed because the cold (to her) weather kept demanding her attention. She had on several layers, including a wool-lined coat. I was in rolled-up shirtsleeves. Herewith the inventory of the only things she said/repeated for a half-hour:

- "It's so cold. I'm all bundled up and you're in shirtsleeves." (At one point I said, "Builds character." She said, "I don't want my character built. I just want to be warm.")
- "Look at all the snow on the mountains." (I gave her many different replies to that, some of which were no reply at all.)
- "You'll have to be patient with me, I just woke up from a sound sleep." (She said that at least ten times, after about six times of which, I couldn't help but ask, "In what sense am I not being patient?"

Her reply, "Well, you just have to be patient with me, I just woke up from a sound sleep.")

- "How was Pam's trip?" (This she asks for the last three days now. She sometimes adds "back east" and I mention that no, it was Hawaii. Then she asks if anyone went with her and I say "all of our kids and their spouses." How many days of this reportage will ensue, I can't foresee.)

That's it. Those four things for about 30 minutes.

The Ugly

Nothing ugly, really. Except this lady in a grungy white van that cut me off in the parking lot.

Dementiadventure 51

Mom's losing steam. Doesn't talk half so much, but repeats herself twice as much. Between the smog and the altitude she labors to get words out, though makes involuntary vocal noises many hours of the day, warding off potential friends at Jamestown.

She won't go outside anymore because of the cold. But she asks how the ducks are surviving. So I take this picture for her: ducks all around the pond with their heads shoved down into their bodies.

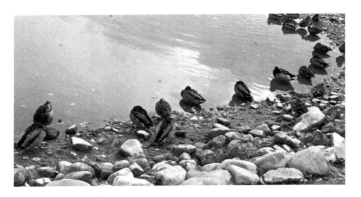

I show it to her and tell her that this is how the ducks try to stay warm. I hope to get a funny reply. But she just says, a few times, "I'm glad I'm not a duck." Then, out of the blue, she says, "I miss California. I miss my old house."

"I know. We all have things we miss." She nods. I ask, "So do you miss any of your husbands?"

She pauses, furrows her forehead. "If I could remember who any of them were, I might."

Dementiadventure 52

Mom's in the hospital. Blood tests show she's massively anemic—her doctor says "Basically, she has no blood"—and CT shows she has a perforated intestine, with pus and air leaking into her belly. The knifing pain in her side and the ravages of infection in her gut have nearly shut her down for good.

We've made some bets on the best course for her and she'll do fine for now with transfusions, antibiotics, and morphine. But no cutting her open. Too much bodily trauma for a little more time at best.

Even so, she's shell-shocked with wires strung to her finger and chest, needles and tubes stuck in both arms. (Her only chuckle of the night is when I ask, "Do you feel like a pin cushion?") Blood-pressure cuff on her bony arm, inflating and deflating on cue every fifteen minutes. Loud beepers going off when a cycle of this or that is done. And the glare everywhere.

"Is all this what's keeping your mom alive?" she asks.

"Pretty much," I say.

"I don't want to spend the rest of my life like this."

"We're just putting you through this until you can come home feeling better."

"Thank you so much for all your help," she says for the fifteenth time or so in the past three hours.

This time I walk over to the machines and monitors, point at them, and say, "Maybe you should be thanking these guys for all *their* help. I'm mostly just hanging around."

She waves at the hardware, pivots her head on the pillow and says, "Thanks, guys." Then, to me, "Is that good enough?"

I think of how she never watches TV at home but how a ceiling-mounted TV always faces you when you're a hospital patient. "Are you going to watch TV while you're here?"

"I don't plan to."

She squirms and groans in the ER bed they've kept her in for half the night. She keeps asking if she'll be able to sleep in her own bed tonight. "No," I keep answering in various ways. "You'll be here for a few nights." Finally, after groggily asking it one last time, she raises a deliberate finger, points at me, and loudly says, "I want you to get me out of this and into my own bed tonight!"

I say, "You can't sleep in your own bed at home tonight, but we'll get you a better bed than this one. This thing's more like a big shopping cart."

"But no one wants to buy me."

Dementiadventure 53

I go to see her this afternoon. She can barely talk. Still, the nurses say, "Marilyn is so funny. Like this morning we were checking on her mental status and asked her if she knew her last name. She said, 'Oh, I've had so many of them.'"

A few other moments from the visit stand out:

- Nature scenes drift across the TV that's hanging from the ceiling. A closeup of a goat's face prompts Mom to say, "Is that me?"
- I'm standing at the foot of her bed and I tell her we're working on getting her out of here and into her own bed at Jamestown. She says, "Yeah, there's not much I can do here but kick your butt."
- I get one of the nurses to put some lip balm on her. As the nurse applies it, Mom says, "Go ahead, make me beautiful. Ha. Ha."
- I tell her that there's not much they can do anymore but try and soothe her pain. "Just shoot me," she says.
  "Well, how about if they shoot you with some more morphine?"
  "Okay. I don't want any more scars."

- "I'm tired of the bed," she says.

  "This bed?"

  "All beds."

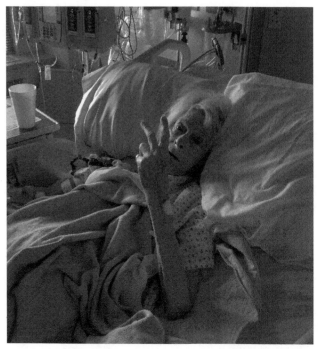

Mom today, looking like your average survivor of Dachau, flashing the peace sign—although the backhand suggests an alternative reference

Dementiadventure 54

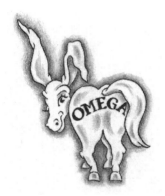

The logo she designed for her San
Jose State sorority, ca. 1947

Doctors are giving Mom five days. She's back in her apartment
junked out on methadone, morphine, Ativan, and one other
one I can't recall. Strange to see a hardy soul slide down so
steeply. She's made her first full-on identity slip that I recall:
her nurse from this morning asked her this afternoon, "Do
you remember me from this morning?" She smiled and said,
"Of course I remember you, Pam."

She's hardly saying anything, really. Her tongue is clotted,
her words slow and slurred. Which means she tries to stick
with good material.

I walk in her bedroom and the first thing she does is point to the wall across from her—where the TV was in the hospital—and says, "A better view."

"Nice to be in your old bed?" I ask.

"My little old bed when I was little? I'd never fit in that one."

"Are you still hurting?"

Long pause. "You didn't kick me or anything, did you?"

"So what are your plans for today?"—I say with a laugh to this woman flat on her back.

She laughs back—a genuine cackle—then points to the ceiling and says, "You better talk to the boss."

In a few minutes I ask her again. "Seriously, what are you going to do today?"

This time she gets more deadpan and says, "I'd like to go out and play football."

"You better not," I say. "You might get hurt."

The nurse comes in with another syringe of methadone and says, "Or hurt someone else."

And I think: *hey, this is my mom's show. No scene stealing.*

Dementiadventure 55

Mom's Last Joke

I always tried to keep her well stocked with the things she used every day—moisturizer, mouthwash, hairspray, floss, toilet paper, tissues, toothpaste, eye drops, lipstick. You'll recall that every time I'd buy her a backup of any of those, she'd say, "I won't live long enough to use all that." I'd give her lots of reasons why that was okay. We could give any leftovers to her friends. We could use them. We could toss them out. It wouldn't matter to her, anyway, I'd tell her, because she'd be gone. When the time came, it would be none of her business.

For eight months she was wrong. She'd run out of something, I'd buy more, and she'd say, again, "I won't live long enough to use all that."

But today she didn't. And the joke's on me. Just the way she'd like it.

Still, she left me a letter, written some years ago, and marked "To be opened upon my death." Here it is, minus the middle paragraph about banks and lawyers:

My Dear Son,

We had some lean years of scrimping while you were growing up, so you may be pleasantly surprised at the amount of your inheritance, much of which is being passed on from your grandfather's hard earned and conservatively accumulated estate. If you invest it wisely, the interest derived from it will reap you a comfortable supplemental income for the rest of your life, as it did for me, and may then be passed on to your children as well. It is my hope that this will be your decision.

Finally, on a more personal note, I am most thankful for having been blessed with you for my son. We had some turbulent years as you were growing up which I truly hope will not all be held to my account, because I, too, was striving to grow up in the process of parenting. You have brought me _much_ pride, and I have loved you dearly although, regretfully, our times together and correspondence have been limited over the years.

My prayer for you is that you and your dear family will remain on a solid foundation, that you will keep the Faith, and that your life will hold much joy along with its inevitable trials and tribulations.

       With abiding love,

          Your Mother

Dementiadventure 56

Passing Notes

The one thing I hadn't thought to think of till now is how Mom's death would hit the other residents of Jamestown.

That "one thing" is actually two things, one small, one big.

The small thing is that people there forget. Some would ask me how Mom was doing, I'd tell them she would be dying soon and in a few minutes, they'd ask the same thing. And I'd answer and each time they were shocked. Choked up, eyes reddening. I had to keep delivering the same blow over and over to these sweet friends.

By the way, I hadn't even known how many friends she had. Most were casual, but all were part of the circle of faces that would glance at each other and nod at every meal, or smile at each other in the halls, or, in my case, have me introduced to them repeatedly for months. My mom liked to eat alone. She'd been assigned to a table of four, but she always took a table for two and lately moved the other chair away so, as she said, she wouldn't have to be chatting with someone she didn't know while she was trying to eat. Still, dozens of people "knew" her, partly for that. And they're missing her now.

The big thing is this: she had two best friends, Evelyn and Marie. Before we moved Mom here, I met Evelyn, who would be her next door neighbor—literally one door two feet from the other. As we moved furniture in for Mom's arrival,

I "met" Evelyn several more times, each time brand new for her. Evelyn hung out exclusively with Marie, a southern belle with a great sense of vocal harmonizing (I've heard her sing a few times with the guy who plays guitar and sings there in the foyer on Sunday afternoons). Once Mom got here, she and they were almost inseparable, too. I virtually never saw one of the trio without at least one of the others a few feet away. Every time I came to visit Mom she would introduce me to Evelyn and/or Marie. In time they seemed to know who I was and who I was there for, though Evelyn thought I was my mom's dad. When I took Mom out for a drive, every third day or so, I always felt bad that I was taking her away from her two friends, who never seemed to have anyone coming to pick them up. They looked sad, not only for Mom leaving them, but that I couldn't take them out, too.

I could go on about these girls and probably have gone on too long already. Let me just say this: Evelyn and Marie are devastated that Mom is gone. They were best friends, hanging out with her every day for eight months. And the only thing worse than seeing them grieve and cry over Mom the last couple of days is the thought that soon, maybe next week, they won't remember her at all. And so the big thing will get folded into the small thing, which happens every day at Jamestown.

Dementiadventure 57

Final Chapter

I went to Jamestown for the last time today, Saturday. Moved the last furniture out, turned in the keys. Mom's best friends Evelyn and Marie were sitting together near the front door, as usual. Evelyn asked me, "How is she?"

I told her, "She passed away on Thanksgiving." She burst into tears.

Marie said, "Was she your wife?"

"No, my mom."

"Oh," she said, nodding. "Your *mom.*"

Together, Pam and I had told Evelyn about Mom's passing six times before.

Mom had introduced me to them both as "my little boy" at least fifty times. But who counts?

Footnote to Dementiadventure

Being with my mom in her last months gave me a new reflex: when someone says "I'll never forget" such and such, I interrupt with "Don't ever say that."

Her Last Diary Entry

It's fashionable to say, "It's the little things." If you ever doubt that, here is my mom's last diary entry, eighty-eight years into this world.

Saturday Sept 12
Busy day — Mike came + got me + we went to big Target store. Also get my dirty purse washed by Pam so didn't need to get a new one. Later in day got my hair washed

Saturday Sept 12
Busy day — Mike came + got me + we went
to big Target store.
Also got my dirty purse washed by Pam so
didn't need to get a new one. Later in day got
my hair washed

November 30

The only drawing of my mom's that hung on her Jamestown wall was this one of her house when she went to San Jose State in the late 1940s. I always asked if we could hang more drawings—no, she said, because she didn't want to put holes in the wall. What about switching this one out with some of her later and better work? No: this one was special because she'd gotten an A+ on it. The only A+ she ever got. I told her grades didn't matter as much as your own opinion of the work.

As you might imagine, we had this conversation a number of times.

I pulled the drawing out of its frame on Saturday, revealing the grade in the bottom right corner. An A. No plus.

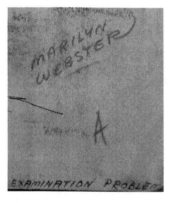

There's a moral or lesson or parable here, I'm sure, but I can't think of it right now. Still, I appreciate the posthumous laugh she gave me.

November 30

I wrote this.

Obituary

Marilyn Frances Thompson
(May 23, 1927–November 26, 2015)

A true California girl, Marilyn Frances Thompson died in Utah on Thanksgiving after a brief illness.

Born on May 23, 1927, she grew up in Santa Paula, amid citrus groves and small storefronts. In the 1930s, her mother taught her art, her father thrift. In the 1940s, including her college years, she drew the eyes of many young men and in 1951 married the first of three husbands, Neil Hicks, with whom she bore her only child, Michael, now an author, composer, and professor. Her third marriage, to Paul Thompson, proved decisive: she knew she'd "finally got it right." (Paul passed away in 1991.)

She lived her life with a spiky mix of grace and stubbornness, truth and beguilement, peace of soul and lip-chewing worry. She loved Jesus, shunned modernism, and resisted the technological deluge of the 1990s and beyond. Yet she found and cultivated her own brand of suburban chic bohemianism in the fiery decades of the 1960s, 1970s, and 1980s—sleek cars, hot pants, record clubs, organic veggies, granola, and always, art: watercolors (in which her mom excelled), acrylics, pencil sketches, pastel and charcoal portraits, pen and ink cartoons, anything that enthused her–or for which she could get paid, which she did till late in her life. She declared herself a "commercial artist" for her death certificate, but also drew maps, proofread, laid out handbooks, kept avid diaries, wrote reams of letters, and mastered all else visible on a page.

Her body will be buried at Alta Mesa Cemetery in Palo Alto, following a brief graveside ceremony at 11 a.m., Friday, December 4, 2015. Flowers welcome but, better still, donate on her behalf to a charity that blesses children.

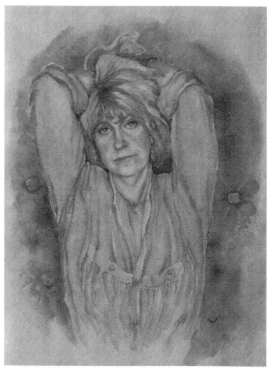

Mom's 1990 watercolor self-portrait, used for the obituary

December 13

So we just held this. Our children were stunning. They and we all, as James Taylor might say, made the roof leak. Here is the talk I gave:

My mom had shelves full of recordings: old 78s from her parents, LPs she got from the record club she belonged to, and 45s she bought at the drugstore. She had records by everyone from Lawrence Welk to Tom Jones, Petula Clark to the Supremes. But I don't remember her ever listening to a single record except one. In 1966, the year she divorced my dad, she came home with a 45 in a nice picture sleeve showing a woman with bleach-blond-teased-and-sprayed hair like her own. It was Dusty Springfield singing "You Don't Have to Say You Love Me." She laid the 7-inch record on the turntable, switched on the power, set the needle down and I heard this French horn start what quickly turned into a huge, ominous orchestral intro sounding like it came from the soundtrack to a murder mystery. And then this husky alto voice started to sing in a minor key:

> When I said I needed you
> You said you would always stay
> It wasn't me who changed but you
> And now you've gone away

After four more lines of this torrid lament, the music suddenly brightened, blossomed like a cactus in the desert, as Ms. Springfield belted out the chorus, now in a major key:

> You don't have to say you love me, just be close
> at hand
> You don't have to stay forever, I will understand
> Believe me, believe me, I can't help but love you
> But believe me I'll never tie you down

My mom played it over and over. Most of the time, you could see her eyes get watery. Sometimes she had to go into her bedroom and close the door for a while.

I said "her bedroom," but I should have said "our bedroom." Because that year she and I, nine years old going on ten, lived in a one-bedroom apartment in South San Jose. Two twin beds with a lighted nightstand between us. One bathroom, of course, where she hung her bras over the shower curtain rod and I threw my jeans in the hamper. A tiny kitchen and living room, where the record player console—one of the few pieces of furniture she got from the divorce—sat against the wall.

I got bussed to fifth and sixth grade each morning—I'd been I.Q.-tested into a special school on the north end of the city—and she went to work at the Gousha company, where she drew illustrations for them—California missions, beach scenes, landscapes and landmarks, whatever a San Jose State commercial art major could muster on demand. After splitting with my dad, and even a little before, she'd started dating other guys. Everywhere she went back then, people told her she looked like Dorothy Malone, the star of *Peyton Place* on TV. She caught the eye of lots of guys, two in particular, one of whom she married during a weekend she left me alone with only Mrs. Figliomeni, the landlady, instructed to check in with me every few hours and make sure I was okay.

I wasn't. My few friends in the neighborhood thought I was stuck up because I went to a special school and my friends at the special school, most of them richer than I'd ever be, couldn't figure out why I didn't know anything. On the way to Mom's divorce I'd found out the three brothers I'd grown up with were only half-brothers, children of dad's first marriage, which I also hadn't known about. The best part of those years was being babysat after school at John Perry's house, where I listened to Herb Alpert and the Tijuana Brass, read *Life* magazines that his parents got, and talked with him about everything from the meaning of women's measurements to why my youngest half-brother was in Vietnam.

Even though I shared a bedroom with her, I thought at the time that Mom was more dutiful than attentive to me. I was a prop and an obligation. Because she needed a man, a full-grown man. Honestly, that was the overriding fact of her whole life, from Jim, her high school sweetheart and first fiancé, to my dad, to the guy she slept with on the way out of that marriage, and then on to her next husband in a marriage that lasted two years, during the latter year of which he never spoke to either Mom or me, but only to his dog about us, in front of us—which was better than him yelling at Mom about me or spanking me, a twelve-year old, like I was the rump of a tired horse. So many boyfriends between marriages, occasionally during marriages, and then in the mid-1970s a boyfriend who provided her one good marriage, the third one, that lasted thirteen years till that truck-driving husband, Paul, died of pneumonia on the way to dying of lung cancer.

Through all this, Mom and I had the kind of relationship that Dusty Springfield song was about. We didn't have to say "I love you." And we didn't. We just had to be close at hand. I wouldn't tie her down and she wouldn't me. Even though I was no boyfriend, I was always her "little boy," as she always called me till the day she died. And for that she could be generous, some might say, to a fault. For instance, when I was in grade school and junior high she took me to drive-in movies with her all the time. I loved horror and sci-fi. So she took me to any of those kinds of movies I wanted to see. We saw *Fantastic Voyage* and *Planet of the Apes* together and, between them, schlocky triple bills of slasher films and worse-than-B-movies like *The Brain that Wouldn't Die*.

Not really having a decent dad put me behind in lots of things. I didn't know about dating, or tying ties, nothing about tools, or cars, or wiring, or plumbing. I did know a lot about art and music, though. Both those things I got from her. She taught me how to draw, always made sure I had crayons or pencils or pastels or ballpoints or even Rapidograph pens in my hands until I went to college. She got me watercolors and acrylics, even fluorescent poster paint in the psychedelic '60s. She showed me how to shade and crosshatch, how to draw life-like eyes and grinning cartoon faces. Meanwhile, at night she played hymns and old standards on our jangly spinet piano. "These Foolish Things," "Talk of the Town," "Fascination," and "Body and Soul," interspersed with "How Great Thou Art," "I Need Thee Every Hour," "Rock of Ages," and "Sweet Hour of Prayer." And I'd imitate her, playing what I could by ear for hours at a time. She bought me LPs, vinyl records that shaped me, from the soundtracks to *Pink Panther* and the *Batman* TV show to headier stuff like the Beatles' *Magical Mystery Tour* and the "White Album." And how's this for not tying me down: she let me go without her or any other adult to see the Doors in concert four days before my twelfth birthday. That was my present.

I said she had lots of records she didn't listen to. She also had lots of books, none of which I saw her read except the daily devotional pamphlets she kept on her nightstand. Oh, and the Bible, of course, from which she taught me verses from the time I was two, when she put me on the pulpit at First Baptist Church in San Jose to recite John 3:16 by heart. If she didn't lead me to books, she did lead me to the Good Book. She loved church almost as much as she loved men, though sometimes it was hard to tell, especially when she'd meet and start dating a man at church, her usual gambit. After the first divorce, she rescued me from that Baptist church into the freestyle Peninsula Bible Church—PBC, as everyone called it—whose new youth minister was the singer-songwriter John Fischer. He was the man who got me to read the modern New Testament translation called *Good News for Modern Man*. He invited me to play guitar in his little Christian garage band, but more important, talked to me about God when he could see I was lonely, drifting into theft and drugs. He got me thinking about art-and-religion for the first time, too. I could give lots of examples, but try this one: John taught a Sunday School class on King Crimson's first album and the meaning of its opening song, "21st Century Schizoid Man." So you see, by Mom's divine sleight-of-hand, she'd brought me into this new kind of faith-world, one where God cares about what we care about and the rest is just cosmic gravy.

All through high school I was a Jesus Freak filing off with my own fellow disciples while she was out, as we'd say at the time, "doing her thing." At night I worked in Christian halfway houses while she went to Parents Without Partners parties and migrated among would-be boyfriends. We never went to church together, though we both went all the time. We weren't close in those days, not even "close at hand," except for living in the same apartment—separate bedrooms now. This is how it was. We kept our doors closed; but we never slammed them. We hardly spoke; but we never yelled at each other. We were a team, just not the same team.

I never knew what was more corrosive to her, her first two marriages or the swinging singles lifestyle between and after them. She could put on a glamour face, groom herself fastidiously, but she often seemed empty and blank-eyed. Valium was part of that. Working long hours in the early days of Silicon Valley was another part, from Hewlett-Packard to Memorex to lots of small vendors scattered around the San Francisco peninsula. She'd often say years later that she wasn't much of a mom to me then and I really don't know what kind of a son I was, except that my bad-boy days of junior high had drowned in the wake of her prayers. The worst thing she ever caught me at in high school was cutting classes to march in an anti-Vietnam war demonstration down University Avenue in Palo Alto. She saw me on the TV news.

We got closer in the mid-1970s. She had a steady boyfriend, I had a steady girlfriend, and we both had steady jobs. She bought a house, a sturdy one-bedroomer in Los Altos, built just after the end of the Second World War. We converted its storeroom into a bedroom for me. It had its own door to the outside, so I'd come and go and not see her sometimes for days.

Still, she liked my girlfriend and I liked her boyfriend, and we'd all do things together sometimes. Then, in the fall of 1974, this song hit the airwaves. It shocked me a bit because it made me think not of me and a girl or me and a friend, but of me and my mom. Helen Reddy sang it:

> You and me against the world
> Sometimes it feels like you and me against the world
> When all the others turn their backs and walk away,
> You can count on me to stay

That's how we both felt. But I couldn't know then what the last lines would come to mean for us:

> And when one of us is gone
> And one of us is left to carry on
> Then remembering will have to do
> Our memories alone will get us through
> Think about the days of me and you
> You and me against the world

As years passed we carved out a typical mom-son long-distance routine. She got married and I got married. Occasional phone calls, cards, visits. She carefully inscribed birthdays and addresses and phone numbers on a huge card next to an antique clock in her breakfast nook. We moved to Illinois, then California again, then Utah. She stayed in her Los Altos house, adding a garish master bedroom on the back, plush red and black with gold trimmings, stocked with exotica that suited her new husband. She set up an in-home studio, too, and moonlighted with piecework for ad hoc clients alongside her day job as a proofreader. She drew cartoons of friends and co-workers and especially Paul. Beyond that, she crafted hundreds of pastel, charcoal, pen, and pencil pictures of dozens of models, including our children, her neighbors, dogs, cats, and dolls. She had to keep her eye-to-hand skills honed. That was who she was, with a man or without. Meanwhile, Pam and I raised four children on a music professor's salary and small envelopes of royalties from books I wrote. I composed music, too, played it, conducted it, recorded it. Mom and I both constructed seemingly useless things incessantly—she with her eyes, me with my ears—both of us obsessed with our quests like addicts. Different veins, same pulse.

When Paul died in 1991, half of her died with him. Other boyfriends came and went. One even travelled the world with her. But all of them—including that second ex-husband, who dallied with her yet again—seemed like merely comfy companionships, lowbrow sequels to the marriage in which, as she said, "I finally got it right." For the last two decades of her life she didn't have a computer or even cable TV, just rabbit ears on a 13-incher. She prided herself on long daily walks. She had a few friends closer at hand than her only child. And for that proximity, some of them might think they knew her better than I. But they would be wrong.

Nevertheless, it doesn't matter. Because by the time she died, halfway into her eighty-ninth year, she couldn't remember anything I've been talking about. None of it. She couldn't even recall that record she once loved, whose third verse went:

> Left alone with just a memory
> Life seems dead and so unreal

When we moved her from her Los Altos home to a group home near us in Utah in the spring of 2015, I knew that the only thing worse than being alone with just a memory was being alone without one. So I decided to do the remembering for both of us. And that was an honor. Because as she got older and older in my eyes and I got younger and younger in hers, I felt our long journey against the world together tumbling through space like a gymnast flying off the uneven bars and all I wanted for us was to stick the landing.

We did.

I've written and posted online lots of adventures of mind and heart she and I undertook in her last eight months. And I could write a thousand times more details of the glories and bitterness of our long, intertwining lives. Let me just say this: in the months before she died, and especially the days before, we did say we loved each other. Lots of times. She wouldn't get to stay forever, that we both understood. But she died knowing that, believe me, believe me, we'd never tied each other down. Not once.

77270778R00064

Made in the USA
Columbia, SC
25 September 2017